Phytochemicals

What You Should Know - A Quick Booklet about Phytonutrients

Sarah Sparrow

PUBLISHED BY:
Sarah Sparrow
Copyright © 2012

All rights reserved.

No part of this publication may be copied, reproduced in any format, by any means, electronic or otherwise, without prior consent from the copyright owner and publisher of this book.

Disclaimer
The information contained in this eBook is for general information purposes only. The information is provided by the authors and while we endeavor to keep the information up to date and correct, we make no representations or warranties of any kind, express or implied, about the completeness, accuracy, reliability, suitability or availability with respect to the eBook or the information, products, services, or related graphics contained in the eBook for any purpose. Any reliance you place on such information is therefore strictly at your own risk.

Table of Contents

Introduction 6
How Phytochemicals Work 6

Most Common Phytochemicals Found in Fruits and Vegetables 7
- Carotenoids 7
- Flavonoids 8
- Sulphoraphane 9
- Limonene 10
- Indoles 10
- Allium Compound 10

Characteristics and Colors of Phytochemicals in Fruits and Veggies 10
- Red 11
- Green 11
- Blue and Purple 12
- Yellow and Orange 13
- White/ Brown/ Tan 13

A to Z of Fruits and Vegetables that are Rich in Phytochemicals 14

Benefits of Phytochemicals 20

Variety Matters 23

Food Processing and Phytochemicals 23

Phytochemicals as Protection from Diseases 24

Introduction

Phytochemicals are bioactive compounds found in natural sources, particularly in plant foods. These elements work with the existing nutrients and fiber in fruits and vegetables to boost the body's immune system to make it resistant to diseases and infections.

Also called phytonutrients, there are different forms of these elements. And each one has its own unique benefits to offer to health-conscious individuals. Characterized mainly by its colors, it is easy to distinguish which types of fruits and vegetables carry a particular form of phytochemical.

How Phytochemicals Work

Filling up one's diet with fruits and vegetables that are rich in phytochemicals lowers the risk of developing chronic diseases like cancer, heart diseases, and diabetes. Its antioxidant properties also help in protecting the body from free radicals in the environment and the food we eat. As cancer-causing agents are deactivated and controlled, you can live a healthier and happier life.

Although there are phytochemical supplements available on the market today, these are not as effective as natural sources. The phytochemicals actually work together with the vitamin and mineral components of food, as well as the dietary fiber that are present in such sources. Supplements lack this special combination, as they offer limited amounts of nutrients. Compounds from natural sources, however, are more readily processed and absorbed by the body.

Most Common Phytochemicals Found in Fruits and Vegetables

Carotenoids

Carotenoids are the pigments which are responsible for such colors as orange, red, green, and yellow. This phytochemical reduces the risk of having heart problems as well as eye problems. Diseases like cancer and diabetes can also be avoided, and the early signs of aging can likewise be controlled. The following compounds belong to this family of phytochemicals:

- **Beta-Carotene** – This brings out the color of orange in fruits and veggies. It slows down the signs of aging, and also aids in the prevention of cancer and diabetes. Some examples of produce that bear this element include mangoes, papaya, apricot, carrots, and pumpkin.

- **Lycopene** – This element brings out the color of red in plant sources. It lowers the risk of developing cancer (particularly prostate cancer) and cardiovascular diseases. Some of the common sources of this phytochemical include pink grapefruit, watermelon, red pepper and tomatoes.

- **Lutein** – This is essential for the maintenance of healthy vision. Cataracts as well as blindness can be avoided when there is sufficient supply of Lutein in the system. You can get this element from crops like spinach, kale, and romaine lettuce.

- **Zeaxanthin** – This compound reduces the risk of cancer and losing one's vision. Food sources include spinach and corn.

Flavonoids

This is another large family of Phytochemicals. As this is an antioxidant, it is a protective substance. By neutralizing and deactivating the unstable molecules inside the body (also called free radicals) you will have a solid defense against diseases like cancer and stroke. Examples of produce that are rich in this compound include oranges, berries, apples, broccoli, and onion. The following elements belong to this group of phytonutrients:

- **Resveratrol** – Aside from lowering the risk of developing cancer and heart diseases, it also aids in proper blood clotting. This element is found in red grapes.

- **Anthocyanins** – This is an effective element against aging. It also improves one's balance and coordination as well as memory as it aids in keeping the nerves and central nervous system healthy. Moreover, it is also helpful in maintaining a healthy urinary tract. You can get this from fruits like strawberries, plums, cranberries, and blueberries.

- **Hesperidin** – This is particularly good for the heart and can help in preventing heart diseases. Citrus fruits like oranges, lemons, and limes are all rich in this compound.

- **Tangeritin** – This is an anti-cancer substance and can help in minimizing cases of tumor around the neck and head area. Citrus fruits such as tangerine, mandarin and oranges all carry this phytonutrient.

- **Quercetins** – Having this type of phytochemical in the body reduces internal inflammation that can result from having allergies. It also inhibits cancer growth particularly on the head and neck areas. Apples, grapes, pears, onions and garlic are all good sources of this element.

Sulphoraphane

This phytochemical reduces the risk of cancer, particularly on the colon. You can get this from food sources like broccoli, kale, Brussel sprouts, and cauliflower.

Limonene

This element reduces the risk of certain cancers (breast, colon, prostate, etc.) and also protects the lungs from the harmful effects of smoking and other pollutants in the air. Citrus fruits like oranges, lemons, limes and grapefruits are all rich in this phytochemical.

Indoles

This compound is an anti-cancer agent. Veggies like broccoli, kale and watercress all have this substance in them.

Allium Compound

This phytochemical is responsible for lowering cholesterol levels as well as regulating the body's blood pressure. Garlic, leeks and onions all have this phytonutrient.

Characteristics and Colors of Phytochemicals in Fruits and Veggies

The colors that you see in the fruits and vegetables that you eat actually signify the types of phytochemicals contained therein. Bright colors of red, orange, yellow and green are just some of the common colors that you see in different crops. Listed below are the different color groups that bear different pigmentation qualities as well as some examples of fruits and veggies.

Red

This color represents the presence of ***Lycopene*** and ***Anthocyanins***. These elements are important in maintaining healthy heart and urinary tract. Furthermore, one's memory will improve significantly when these phytochemicals are always included in the diet.

- Red Apples
- Red Peppers
- Strawberries
- Cranberries
- Raspberries
- Watermelon
- Pomegranates

Green

Fruits and veggies that are colored green are rich in ***Lutein*** and ***Indoles***. These phytochemicals help prevent cancer, and aids in bone and teeth health as well.

- Green Apple
- Avocados

- Lime
- Asparagus
- Artichokes
- Broccoli
- Brussels Sprouts
- Cucumber
- Lettuce
- Spinach

Blue and Purple

Fruits and veggies that bear this type of color signify high amounts of **Phenolics** and **Anthocyanins**. Because of its antioxidant properties, this element contributes to the prevention of cancer and controls the aging process as well. Research also shows that it aids in alleviating the symptoms of urinary tract infection.

- Grapes
- Blackberries
- Blueberries
- Plums

- Purple Cabbage
- Eggplant

Yellow and Orange

Aside from having vitamin C contents, produce that bear these colors also carry **_Carotenoids_** and **_Bioflavonoids_**. These phytochemicals are essential to heart and vision health, and they also strengthen the immune system so as to make it resistant to serious diseases like cancer and cardiovascular problems.

- Oranges
- Grapefruits
- Apricots
- Mangoes
- Lemon
- Papaya
- Pineapples
- Carrots

White/ Brown/ Tan

Crops with these colors contain **_Allicin_** which is known for its benefits to the heart.

- Bananas
- Dates
- Onion
- Garlic
- Cauliflower
- Ginger
- Mushroom

A to Z of Fruits and Vegetables that are Rich in Phytochemicals

As fruits and vegetables are the best sources of phytonutrients, it is important to know which types of produce carry a particular form of compound. Listed below are some of the best crops that are readily available on the market. You can consume these in order to benefit from its phytochemical components.

1. **Apples** – This fruit contains *Quercetin* which helps prevent asthma attacks and complications of diabetes. It also carries *Phenolic compound* which is essential for a healthy heart.

2. **Apricots** – As a fruit that's rich in *Beta-Carotene*, this is both anti-aging and anti-cancer.

3. **Blackberries** – Carrying the phytochemical *Ellagic Acid*, this fruit helps in regulating the body's cholesterol levels.

4. **Blueberries** – Containing *Anthocyanins*, this element helps in reversing the signs of aging. Its *Ellagic Acid* contents also give it anti-cancer properties.

5. **Bok Choy** – This veggie carries a lot of phytochemicals including *Sulphoraphane* and *Indoles* which are both anti-cancer.

6. **Broccoli** – This vegetable is one of the most nutritious crops as it carries a number of vitamins, minerals and phytochemicals. It has *Sulphoraphane*, *Indoles*, *Beta-Carotene*, and *Lutein*. All these elements contribute to eye and lung health, and they are also anti-cancer and anti-aging.

7. **Brussels Sprouts** – As one of the biggest carriers of *Sulphoraphane*, this works against carcinogenic substances which can lead to cancer.

8. **Cabbage** – Containing both *Sulphoraphane* and *Indoles*, this is a great anti-cancer veggie.

9. **Cantaloupe** – The *Beta-Carotene* component of this produce makes it helpful to people suffering from diabetes and cancer. It also has

anti-aging properties and can contribute to having healthy lungs.

10. **Cauliflower** – This vegetable contains 2 types of phytochemicals, namely, *Sulphoraphane* and *Indoles*. These are cancer-fighting agents.

11. **Cherries** – Rich in *Anthocynanins*, this fruit carries anti-aging properties. Its *Quercetin* component also makes it anti-inflammatory, and is especially helpful to those with allergies.

12. **Corn** – This crop bears *Zeaxanthin* which can help prevent many types of visual impairment including macular degeneration. When not properly monitored, this condition can lead to blindness.

13. **Garlic** – This veggie which is commonly used in all types of recipes contains *Allium compound*, which is anti-cancer. It also aids in regulating proper levels of cholesterol and blood pressure. Its *Quercetin* content also helps in reducing symptoms of inflammation which are associated with allergic reactions.

14. **Kale** – Containing high levels of *Beta-Carotene*, this phytochemical helps in protecting the lungs from suffering heavy damages that may be caused by smoking cigarettes. It also carries *Lutein* which is known for its benefits to the eye health.

15. **Leeks** – With high levels of *Allium compounds*, this helps in promoting normal levels of cholesterol and blood pressure.

16. **Lettuce** – This type of leafy vegetable carries *Quercetins* which can increase the body's resistance against inflammation caused by allergies. This phytochemical is also anti-cancer and can help in preventing the growth of tumors especially on the head and neck areas.

17. **Mangoes** – This is one of the fruits that contain high amounts of *Beta-Carotene*. This is essential in keeping the lungs and heart healthy. It is also anti-aging and anti-cancer.

18. **Onions** – The *Allium compounds* in this veggie is good for the heart, and it also aids in keeping a normal blood pressure. Its *Quercetin* components, on the other hand, help in fighting off inflammation due to allergic reactions.

19. **Oranges** – This citrus fruit carries *Hesperidin* and *Tangeritin* which both serve as antioxidants. Heart diseases as well as cancer can be avoided when sufficient amounts of these phytochemicals are supplied to the body. Its *Limonene* components also aid in protecting the lungs from the harmful effects of smoking.

20. **Papaya** – As its color suggests, this fruit is rich in *Beta-Carotene*. This slows down the aging

process, and also helps in protecting the lungs from pollutants.

21. **Pears** – The *Quercetin* content of this type of fruit helps in maintaining strong and well-functioning lungs.

22. **Pink Grapefruit** – The *Lycopene* component in this citrus fruit is responsible in keeping the body resistant to certain forms of cancer (prostate, breast, etc). Having antioxidant phytochemicals like *Hesperidin* and *Tangeritin* also aid in avoiding heart diseases.

23. **Plums** – Having *Anthocyanins*, this helps in slowing down the signs and early symptoms of aging.

24. **Prunes** – As a source of *Phenolic compounds*, loss of memory can be avoided and one's learning ability is also enhanced.

25. **Pumpkin** – By supplying the body with *Beta Carotene*, the system is made stronger to fight off chronic diseases like cancer and stroke.

26. **Raisins** – As *Phenolic compounds* have antioxidants properties, it can slow down the aging process both inside and out.

27. **Raspberries** – The *Allegic Acid* present in this type of fruit is an anti-cancer agent, and it helps in controlling one's cholesterol levels too.

28. **Red Grapes** – Containing *Resveratrol*, this makes this type of fruit contributory to controlling and alleviating heart problems.

29. **Red Peppers** – As the color of red signifies high *Lycopene* components, this helps in controlling the development of certain types of cancer (e.g. prostate, colon, etc.).

30. **Romaine Lettuce** – The *Lutein* content of this leafy veggie aids in keeping the eye healthy so as to avoid having cataracts and other eye problems that can lead to blindness.

31. **Spinach** – This veggie is a powerhouse of vitamins, minerals, and phytochemicals. It contains *Beta-Carotene*, *Lutein*, and *Zeaxanthin* which aid in slowing the natural process of aging and helps in the prevention of cancer as well.

32. **Strawberries** – This red-colored fruit is rich in *Ellagic Acid*, and it helps in lowering bad cholesterol levels.

33. **Sweet Potatoes** – Containing high *Beta-Carotene* component aids in keeping the lungs healthy, and in preventing cancer too.

34. **Squash** – This veggie contains *Zeaxanthin*, and it helps in avoiding eye problems like macular degeneration and cataract.

35. **Tomatoes** – This is one of the richest sources of *Lycopene*. Cardiovascular diseases as well as cancer can be avoided when the diet has ample supply of this phytochemical.

36. **Watercress** – Its *Sulphoraphane* content gives this crop its anti-cancer properties.

37. **Watermelon** – As a rich source of *Lycopene*, certain types of cancer (breast, prostate, colon, etc.) as well as heart problems can be avoided.

Benefits of Phytochemicals

Phytochemicals in food, particularly in fresh fruits and vegetables, are equally important as the vitamin and mineral contents of said food sources. In fact, all these elements work together in keeping the body strong and healthy. Here's a breakdown of the advantages of supplying the body with natural bioactive compounds.

1. **Slows Down the Aging Process** – As the body is supplied with essential nutrients, it can cope better with the natural process of aging. The organs function well, so as to detoxify the body naturally from the inside. This is manifested by feeling young and looking young as well.

2. **Heart Problems are avoided** – Heart diseases that can lead to cardiac arrest can be avoided as the organ is nourished and strengthened.

3. **Cancer Prevention** – As phytochemicals also work as antioxidants, it lessens the risk of acquiring certain types of cancer (breast, colon, prostate, etc). Free radicals that are present in one's environment are deactivated, and the body's immune system is strengthened to make it more resistant against such a deadly disease.

4. **Controls Eye Diseases** – Foods that are rich in natural compounds assist in maintaining eye health so as not to lose vision as one grows old. Macular degeneration as well as cataracts can be avoided when sufficient vitamins, minerals, and phytochemicals are supplied to the body regularly.

5. **Lowers Risk of Osteoporosis** – Phytochemicals are also contributory to bone health. Aside from the calcium content in certain types of food, its reaction to the compounds make it more effective in maintaining strong bones as the demand for its maintenance increases with age.

6. **UTI Prevention**– The anti-bacterial properties of phytonutrients help the body become more resistant to infections of the urinary tract.

7. **Defense against Colds and Flu** – Phytochemical compounds also carry anti-virus properties, and this increases the body's resistance against viral infections.

8. **Assists in Lung Health** – Certain phytochemicals are especially good for the lungs as it strengthens this organ so that it can cope with the poisonous elements in the environment.

9. **Regulates Blood Pressure** – As the bioactive compounds work with other nutritious substances inside the body, all internal organs start to function properly thereby promoting normal blood pressure.

10. **Controls Symptoms of Diabetes** – The chemical composition of phytochemicals work with vitamins and minerals to regulate the body's sugar levels. This helps in avoiding the progression of diabetes and its complications as well.

11. **Maintains Normal Cholesterol Levels** – The presence of phytochemicals increases the efficiency of the vitamins, minerals, and live enzymes that are contained in food sources.

12. **Hormone Metabolism** – Phytochemical compounds promote the right balance of

hormones inside the body to help reduce anxiety attacks and mood swings.

13. **For Detoxification Purposes** – Because of the antioxidant properties contained in phytochemicals, the body's internal organs are naturally detoxified of harmful substances and toxic elements.

14. **Stronger Immune System** – The combination of phytochemicals, vitamins, minerals, and live enzymes all help in building up and boosting the body's immune system so as to make it more resistant to different forms of diseases.

Variety Matters

Each fruit and vegetable color group has its own unique benefits, and consuming a wide variety of produce will provide the body with hundreds of phytochemicals, vitamins, and minerals. In order to get optimum results, you can generally consume one cup of each of the different color groups in a day. Five to nine servings is recommended, as this will ensure that you are getting a wide source of nutrients and phytochemicals in your diet.

Food Processing and Phytochemicals

The phytochemicals that are present in fresh food sources are easily destroyed by preparation techniques like cooking and processing. When this happens, the body will benefit from fewer forms of phytochemicals and other nutritious substances that could otherwise be present in such sources of food. As these compounds are necessary for good health, one's general state is put at risk. The body is exposed to acquiring simple ailments like colds and flu, and even chronic diseases like cancer, diabetes and heart problems.

Phytochemicals as Protection from Diseases

In spite of its scientific name, phytochemicals are not made from artificial and harmful chemicals. These are natural sources of nutrients that can make the body stronger and more resistant to germs and microorganisms through daily consumption.

Fruits and vegetables are its best sources, and you can even choose the type of phytonutrients that are most beneficial to your condition as these are color-coded. You should know that the brighter the colors of the produce, the higher the amounts of phytochemicals that are contained therein.

Scientific research has shown that these bioactive compounds are effective and safe. And daily consumption of the recommended dosage can improve one's general health.

Printed in Great Britain
by Amazon